# THE
# WARRIOR'S
# MIND

**First Edition – 2025**

Published by **Lead From Within**
LeadFromWithin.co

ISBN - 979-8-218-80748-1
ebook ISBN - 979-8-218-80749-8
**Published in the United States of America**

For permissions or inquiries, contact:
**adam@leadfromwithin.co**

# How to Use This Book

This book is built around 9 chapters, each one a step forward on your journey. Inside, you'll find personal stories, structured exercises, deep reflection prompts, and open journal spaces to help you explore what you're feeling.

Start by reading it from beginning to end, letting each chapter guide you in its own way. Then, revisit the sections that resonate most —especially on the hard days—to recenter yourself and draw strength.

This isn't a book you read once and put away. It's a companion you can return to whenever you need clarity, focus, or a reminder of the progress you've already made.

# INTRODUCTION

## MY JOURNEY WITH ANXIETY:
### *A PERSONAL STORY*

I've dealt with stress and anxiety from an early age, starting my journey to overcome these challenges at just 12 years old. Being diagnosed with anxiety wasn't easy. It took **trials and tribulations** to overcome these a day at a time, while adapting to a different way of coping with anxiety. There was a period of being **homeschooled** during middle school. I missed out essentially on most of my middle school and high school years from the end of 6th grade to my sophomore year in high school. Over the years, I've worked hard to **strengthen** my **mind, body, and spirit**, becoming more open to understanding the world around me. Through this process, I've learned to **live with optimism,** connect deeply with others, and even help people in ways I never imagined—sometimes without even realizing it.

# MY JOURNEY WITH ANXIETY:
## A PERSONAL STORY CONTINUED

One of the most defining moments in my life came when my parents separated when I was 19. I suddenly found myself **balancing the emotional weight** of supporting both my mother and father while also being a role model for my younger brother. It was an **overwhelming challenge** that tested me in ways I wasn't prepared for. At times, I resented life and felt **consumed by anxiety**. But through that struggle, I discovered resilience within myself that I didn't know existed.

That experience taught me to appreciate what I have and shaped me into the **person I am today**—independent, mentally resilient, and deeply grateful for life's lessons. Along the way, I've achieved milestones in my family that no one before me has reached, filling me with a sense of pride that's truly priceless. Looking back now, **I wouldn't change** a thing because every challenge brought me closer to understanding myself and my purpose.

# WHY GUIDANCE IS NECESSARY
## EVEN WHEN IT'S NOT VISIBLE

Seeking guidance isn't a weakness— it's a tool that strengthens the ability to overcome anxiety.
Many men, and people in general, struggle with anxiety in silence, often feeling the pressure to figure things out alone. The presence of guidance, invisible guidance, will act as an anchor to help navigate challenges.

### What is invisible guidance?

1.  **Subconscious Influence** – The lessons we absorb over time shape our reactions to anxiety, even when we don't realize it.
2.  **Emotional Blueprint** – Past role models leave an imprint on how we handle stress and uncertainty.
3.  **Cultural & Social Conditioning** – The beliefs we inherit guide our decisions, making it essential to choose healthy influences.
4.  **Self-Guidance Through Internalized Wisdom** – Over time, external advice becomes our inner voice, helping us navigate challenges.
5.  **Unseen Support Systems** - Friends, family, and communities provide quiet but crucial emotional support.

## The Three Pillars:

### 1. Navigating the Mindset
Chapters 1-3

### 2. Showing Vulnerability and Openness
Chapters 4-6

### 3. Accepting your Emotions
Chapters 7-9

# CHAPTER ONE

# UNDERSTANDING ANXIETY & MASCULINITY

**Key Message:** *Anxiety doesn't make you weak. It's a signal, not a failure.*

I've often internalized anxiety, letting my thoughts spiral into worst-case scenarios and endless "what ifs." It's not just uncomfortable—it feels like you're trapped with no way out. But taking a step back can make a difference. Pause and assess the situation. Acknowledge the "what ifs" and challenge them instead of letting them control you. Use breathing techniques, like the **Navy SEAL method**:

Inhale for 3 seconds – Hold for 3 seconds – Exhale for 3 seconds- Hold for 3 seconds. (Repeat 5-10 times.)

Even if you don't fully understand why you're anxious, recognizing and naming the feeling is a win. Awareness is the first step to regaining control.

# Personal Reflection: When Anxiety Hits Out of Nowhere

There have been moments—out of nowhere—when I'd be on my way to work and suddenly start hyperventilating. Everything would've been fine just minutes before. No warning, no obvious trigger. And suddenly, I'm questioning how I even got to that point. My mind would spiral into what-ifs—racing from worst-case to best-case scenarios like a mental rollercoaster. The frustration would hit hard. I'd have to stop whatever I was doing and just shut down for a moment.

But here's what I learned to do: I talked myself through it. I reminded myself that I've been here before, and I made it through. I told myself, "This is doable. I'm not alone. I'm strong mentally. I just need to give five minutes back to ME."

That small pause—those five minutes—helped me regain control. They reminded me that I'm the priority. Choosing to reclaim power over my thoughts shifted something in me. Over time, those small moments built up into a surge of confidence.

**Here's what I want you to take from this:**

Don't be hard on yourself. We all have our days.
It's not easy in the moment, but on the other side of it, you'll realize —you made it.
And you'll know you can do it again.
Keep going. You're stronger than you think.

# Structured Exercise:

1. List three common beliefs about masculinity and emotions.

2. Rate each belief (1-5) based on how much it has influenced you.

3. Rewrite **ONE** belief in a way that promotes your emotional health. HOW HAS THIS MADE YOU STRONGER? *EX: "I know that where I am today is a blessing compared to where I was yesterday. Yesterday was rough and full of difficult moments, but today I've learned, grown, and pushed through. I'm standing stronger now than I was before. I've taken time to appreciate the progress I've made, and I'm continuing to build the mental resilience I need to keep moving forward."*

# Deep Reflection Prompts:

Think about a time when you felt pressure to "man up" aka suppress your emotions. Think about *"When Anxiety Hits Out of Nowhere."*

• What was the situation?

• How did you respond?

• How might you have handled it differently?

# Daily Journal

YOUR THOUGHTS

Date:

My Thoughts Today:

My Goals:

# CHAPTER TWO

# REFRAMING NEGATIVE THOUGHTS

**Key Message:** *Your thoughts shape your reality, but you have the power to reshape them.*

Men often internalize **negative thoughts**, leading to self-doubt, avoidance, or even emotional shutdown. Reframing is about challenging automatic negative thoughts (**ANTs**) and replacing them with more balanced, constructive perspectives. All of the "I don't, I'm not, what if, and maybe this isn't me," mental blocks that cross our minds each day are challenging. Recognizing, challenging, and **replacing these thoughts** will reframe the negative thought process and turn it into something even greater.

# THE PROCESS OF REFRAMING

**1.** Recognize the Negative Thought

- **Example:** *"I'm not good enough for this job."*

**2.** Challenge It with Logic

- Ask yourself: *"Is this 100% true? What proof do I have?"*
- **Example:** "I got the interview, so they clearly see potential in me."

**3.** Replace It with a Constructive Thought

- Instead of: *"I always mess up."*
- **Reframe:** *"I make mistakes, but I learn and improve."*

*When you shift your perspective, you take control instead of letting fear dictate your actions. Over time, this habit strengthens your confidence and emotional resilience.*

# Structured Exercise:

1. Write down a recurring anxious thought.

2. List three pieces of evidence that challenge this thought.

3. Rewrite the thought in a more balanced, constructive way.

**Negative Thought:** "I always mess up."

**Evidence Against It:** "I've handled tough situations before."

**Reframed Thought:** "I make mistakes, but I also grow from them."

# Now it's your turn

**Negative Thought:**

**Evidence Against It:**

**Reframed Thought:**

# Deep Reflection Prompts:

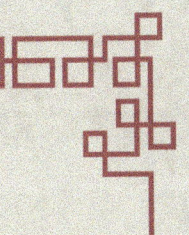

Describe a situation where you assumed the worst but later realized things weren't as bad as they seemed.

• What lesson can you take from that experience?

# Daily Journal

YOUR THOUGHTS

Date:

My Thoughts Today:

My Goals:

# CHAPTER THREE

# STRENGTH AND ADAPTING

**Key Message:** Strength isn't about avoiding struggle—it's about adapting to it.

Have you ever experienced a change—at home, at work, or even during your daily routine—that completely threw you off? Change disrupts the norms we're used to, forcing us to **adapt or resist**. The truth is, change can be beneficial—**if you choose to adapt.**

Recognizing change, accepting your current reality, and using it as a tool for growth sets you up for future success. Struggles—whether mental or physical—aren't roadblocks; they're opportunities to build strength. Instead of running from discomfort, lean into it. Growth happens when you face challenges head-on.

**Resilience isn't about avoiding difficulty**—it's about **learning** to **navigate** it. Embrace the process, and it will shape you into someone **stronger, wiser,** and more **capable**.

# Personal Reflection: When I Chose to Bet on Myself

Thinking back to a big turning point in my life, it was when **I left a job** I had only been in for about **three months**. I was excited—this new path was in music, **something I've always loved.** But leaving my stable "day job" to pursue it full-time? That scared the life out of me.

For the first time, I was calling the shots. I was in charge of how much I made, when I worked, and what I put into the world. The freedom was exciting—but also **overwhelming**. Dealing with a demanding workload and a tough boss made the transition even harder.

**So why did I leave**? Simple: I wasn't getting paid on time. No matter how passionate you are, your work has to sustain you—and waiting for overdue payments while living off savings was stressful. I started job hunting again, determined not to settle just anywhere, especially with the experience I had.

The feeling of **defeat** was **heavy**. But what **helped me adapt** and stay grounded was shifting my mindset. Instead of focusing on fear, doubt, and scarcity, I reminded myself: I had taken control. No one else. That meant I could do it again.

I **kept moving forward**, even on the days when motivation was low. And within a month, I was working again—two jobs. I returned to my old workplace while continuing to pursue my passion. That chapter taught me a lot.

**Here's what I want you to take from this:**

Life will throw you curveballs, but if you keep showing up—even when everything feels off—you'll find your footing. The setbacks become your fuel.

# Structured Exercise:

1. Identify three past challenges you've overcome.

2. What qualities helped you get through them?

3. How can you apply those strengths to current struggles?

# Deep Reflection Prompts:

• What does mental resilience mean to you?

• How can you build it without feeling like you have to suppress emotions?

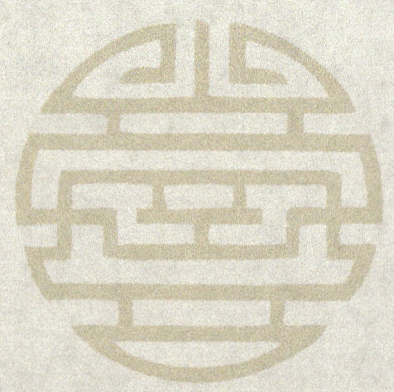

# Daily Journal

Date: _____

My Thoughts Today: _____

My Goals: _____

# CHAPTER FOUR

# THE STRENGHTH IN VULNERABILITY

**Key Message:** Vulnerability is courage, not weakness.

Asking for help and expressing your emotions isn't easy. In fact, **hiding how you feel often seems like the easier option.** But bottling it up only adds to the weight you're carrying.

Vulnerability isn't weakness—it's a step toward **relief and growth.** Letting go of what's inside helps ease the tension of what you're battling. I know this firsthand. It took me years to fully open up to the right person I could trust, and even now, it's something I continue to work on.

Whether you're facing **anxiety, doubt, fear, or just a tough day**, expressing it makes coping easier. The more you allow yourself to be open, the lighter the burden becomes. **Strength isn't in silence—it's in facing what's real.**

# Personal Reflection: Vulnerability is SEXY

For a long time, opening up wasn't easy for me. Admitting how I felt—especially to myself—was one of my biggest challenges. I used to avoid it by staying busy with habits that felt safe. I'd hit the gym, make music, or go for a walk—anything to shift the energy and find some balance.

These things helped, but what really moved the needle was allowing myself to be honest about what I was feeling. Whether it was talking to someone I trust or just sitting with the discomfort, choosing to be vulnerable felt unfamiliar—but powerful.

Because here's the truth: vulnerability isn't weakness. It takes strength to show up raw and real. And that kind of strength? That's what's truly sexy.

# Structured Exercise:

1. Identify three fears about being open with others.

2. What's the worst that could happen?

3. What's the best that could happen?

4. Write down one small step you can take to open up more.

# Deep Reflection Prompts:

Describe a time when you hid your true feelings.

• How did it affect you?

• How might things have changed if you had expressed yourself?

# Daily Journal

Date:

My Thoughts Today:

My Goals:

# CHAPTER FIVE

# EXPRESSING YOURSELF WITHOUT FEAR

**Key Message:** The right people will respect your emotions, not judge them.

Having the right people around you—those you can trust, open up to, and be fully yourself with—makes all the difference. They don't have to be family; they can be close friends, a mentor, a coworker, or even a therapist. What matters is knowing **you're heard without judgment**. Trust creates **comfort, confidence, and authenticity.** When you feel safe, you're more willing to express yourself without holding back. Fear only limits what you can accomplish, keeping you stuck in your own head. The key is to **push past that hesitation and just go for it.** It's not always easy, but with the right support, it's absolutely possible. **Your voice matters—use it.**

# Structured Exercise:

1. Write down three people you trust.

2. What topics feel safest to discuss with them?

3. What's one thing you'd like to share but haven't?

# Deep Reflection Prompts:

What's holding you back from being more open?

• Is it fear, past experiences, or something else?

• What's one step you can take to break this barrier?

# Daily Journal

YOUR THOUGHTS

Date:

My Thoughts Today:

My Goals:

# CHAPTER SIX

# BUILDING A SUPPORT SYSTEM

**Key Message:** You don't have to do this alone.

Why do you even need a support system, and how do you build one?

When we talked about **expressing yourself without fear**, we touched on the power of being open with others. This is the next step—**finding the right people to lean on.**

Even one person who holds you accountable and shows up for you can make a huge difference. If you have a group of friends, seek out those you can truly trust and build your support system around them. The goal isn't just having people around—it's having people who listen, challenge, and support you without judgment.

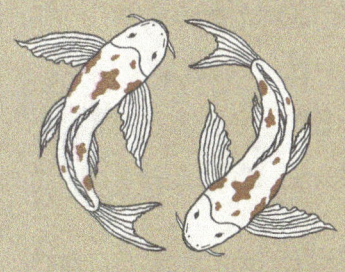

# A STRONG SUPPORT SYSTEM CAN...

✓ *Give you perspective* when your thoughts feel overwhelming.

✓ **Offer advice** or simply be a listening ear.

✓ **Make struggles easier to unpack** so they don't feel as heavy.

If you don't have that support yet, **you're not alone.** There are online groups, local communities, and mentors who have walked this path before you. Some people are in the same boat, looking for connection, while others have been where you are and can **help push you forward** into a stronger, more confident version of yourself.

**Growth happens when you surround yourself with the right energy.** Challenging yourself to build a support system will **boost your confidence, strengthen your mindset, and improve your overall well-being.** You don't have to do it alone—**you just have to take the first step.**

# Personal Reflection: Who is My Support System?

For years, my mom, dad, and brother were the only ones who truly knew what I was dealing with. Letting them in—allowing them to support me—wasn't easy at first. But once I did, it helped shift my perspective. I realized I didn't have to carry everything alone. Just having someone to listen made a huge difference.

Over time, I learned that real connection, with people I trusted, was even more powerful.

Eventually, my support system grew. I found close friends I could open up to, and I trusted my gut in knowing who felt safe. No one's here to judge. We all have our own struggles, and being real about that can create a strong bond.

When you open up, you not only help yourself—you give others permission to do the same. That kind of support can be life-changing

# Structured Exercise:

1. List three qualities of a strong support system.

2. Do you have people who fit these qualities?
   If not, where can you find them?

3. Write down one action step to strengthen your support network.

# Deep Reflection Prompts:

Think about a time when someone supported you.

- How did it feel?

- How can you allow more of that into your life?

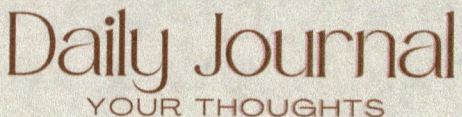

# Daily Journal
YOUR THOUGHTS

Date:

My Thoughts Today:

My Goals:

# CHAPTER SEVEN

# IT'S OKAY TO FEEL THIS WAY

**Key Message:** Emotions don't define you, but ignoring them does more harm than good.

Holding back your emotions, masking how you feel, and resisting growth **only does more harm than good.** Growth takes time, and the first step is **accepting that your emotions are valid.**
What you're going through right now **matters.** Your story, your struggles, and your feelings aren't just yours—someone else out there is facing something similar. **By acknowledging your emotions, you not only help yourself heal but also create space for others to do the same.**
I've learned firsthand that being open to what others are going through has helped me better understand my own challenges. It reminded me that I'm not alone —and neither are you.
Let your emotions be heard, **but don't let them define you**. Feelings are temporary, and every challenge you face is an opportunity to grow. Without struggle, there's no progress. **Embrace what you feel, knowing it's a stepping stone—not a stopping point.**
**It's okay to feel this way. It's part of the process. And you will come out stronger.**

# Personal Reflection:

Recently, I went through an entire week—Sunday to Saturday—where anxiety hit me out of nowhere. It caught me off guard. I hadn't felt it that strongly in a long time, and I kept asking myself, Why is this happening? Where is this coming from? I felt doubt creeping in. There was pressure in my chest, a tightness I couldn't shake. I started questioning everything—even how far I've come on this journey. But then I caught myself. I paused and reminded myself: Look how far you've come.
The following Monday, I made a decision. I set an intention to reclaim my peace. Even though I had a full day ahead, I permitted myself to slow down. When my body began to relax, I told myself, It's okay to feel this way.
Just acknowledging that helped me regain my confidence and mental strength. That week taught me that anxious moments are temporary—and that I don't have to have everything figured out. Focusing on one moment at a time was enough.
Letting go of the need to control the whole day—or the whole week—helped me adapt, and reminded me of my own resilience.

# Structured Exercise: ✳

1. List five emotions you've felt this week.

2. For each, write how you responded to it.

3. Was your response healthy? If not, what could you try next time?

# Deep Reflection Prompts:

Describe a time you fought against your emotions instead of accepting them.

- What was the outcome?

- How might things have changed if you had embraced how you felt?

# Daily Journal

Date:

My Thoughts Today:

My Goals:

# CHAPTER EIGHT

# ANXIETY AS A "TEACHER"

**Key Message:** You don't need to "get rid" of anxiety—you need to work with it.

If there were a way to completely get rid of anxiety, we'd live in a perfect world. But the truth is, **growth doesn't come from avoiding challenges—it comes from learning to navigate them.**
Anxiety can be unpredictable. It can hit first thing in the morning, creep in during the day, or keep your mind racing at night. I've experienced this firsthand—feeling fine one moment, then suddenly overwhelmed the next. It's frustrating, exhausting, and sometimes feels out of your control.
But when I stopped trying to silence it and started listening to it, I realized anxiety was teaching me something. It was showing me where my fears lived. It was exposing the areas where I lacked trust in myself. And most importantly, it was pointing me toward the very challenges I needed to face if I wanted to grow.

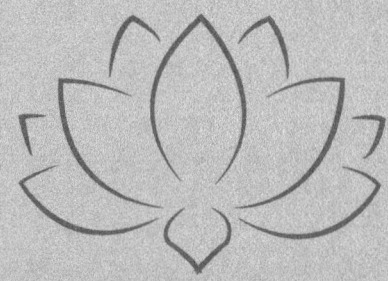

# ANXIETY TEACHES US IN SUBTLE BUT POWERFUL WAYS:

**Anxiety teaches us** in subtle but powerful ways:

- **It tests patience** and forces us to slow down.

- **It reveals triggers,** showing what matters most to us.

- **It builds awareness**, pushing us to look deeper at our habits, thoughts, and beliefs.

- **It teaches resilience,** because every time you face it instead of hiding, you prove to yourself that you can.

**Suppressing anxiety** only creates pressure that eventually bursts. But acknowledging it—sitting with it, journaling about it, breathing through it—transforms anxiety into insight. You begin to recognize patterns, discover what strengthens or weakens you, and **learn** healthier **ways to respond**.

# Structured Exercise:

1. Write down a recent anxious moment.

2. What did you do in the moment?

3. What are three alternative ways to respond that could help next time?

# Deep Reflection Prompts:

What's one habit you have that makes your anxiety worse?

• How can you replace it with something healthier?

# Daily Journal

YOUR THOUGHTS

Date:

My Thoughts Today:

My Goals:

# CHAPTER NINE

# TURNING ANXIETY INTO A STRENGTH

**Key Message:** Anxiety isn't just an obstacle—it can be fuel for growth.

I've had my share of anxiety attacks, and for a long time, I let them control me. But when I started **facing them head-on,** I realized I could navigate through the storm and even use that anxious energy to **push forward,** not pull back. I began treating anxiety like a **superpower**—something I could harness instead of something that held me back.

Anxiety can feel like being trapped in a metaphorical box, but you **don't have to stay there**. The key is to face it, not run from it. In the beginning, it was uncomfortable—**really uncomfortable**. But over time, I realized that every time I confronted my anxiety, I came out **stronger, more confident, and at peace**.

So don't let anxiety **set you back**. Instead, **use it as momentum** to build confidence, resilience, and a better version of yourself. **It's not about avoiding the storm—it's about learning to navigate through it.**

# REDIRECTING ANXIETY INTO ENERGY:

✓ **Journaling** - Putting your thoughts on paper helps you process emotions instead of bottling them up.

✓ **Meditation & Breathing Techniques** - Methods like the Navy SEAL breathing technique (4-4-4) can bring instant calm. Inhale for 4 seconds. Hold that breath for 4 seconds. Exhale for 4 seconds. Hold again for 4 seconds. Now repeat six to ten times.

✓ **Physical Activity** - Working out, going for a walk, or engaging in creative outlets like music or art can help release built-up energy.

✓ **Lean on Your Support System** - Talking with trusted friends, mentors, or therapists can help shift your perspective.

Anxiety doesn't define you, and it doesn't have to control you. **Each time you acknowledge it and face it head-on, you build resilience.** Growth isn't about never feeling anxious—it's about **handling it in a way that makes you stronger.**

# Structured Exercise:

1. Identify one area where anxiety actually helps you (e.g., motivation, awareness).

2. What's one way you can turn anxious energy into something productive?

3. Write down one new coping strategy to try this week.

# Deep Reflection Prompts:

Think about a time when you pushed through anxiety and succeeded.

• What did you learn from that experience?

• How can you remind yourself of that strength when future anxiety arises?

# Daily Journal

YOUR THOUGHTS

Date:

My Thoughts Today:

My Goals:

# From Me to You

I'm proud of you.

You've made it this far—and that means something. You're walking away with more than just tools for yourself; **you're creating a ripple effect** for those around you. This journey isn't a race or a competition—it's a marathon we're all running, side by side, learning how to lift each other up.

I know it's not easy to open up. Letting others in and admitting what you're going through **takes courage** that most people can't see. There were many times I **wished I had a guide** like this during my own darkest moments. But without those struggles, there wouldn't be this story to share—or the one you're now writing for yourself.

**You are not alone in this.**

You have my support, always.

Let's **keep growing**, **keep showing up**, and **keep passing the baton** to the next man who needs it.

"Strong doesn't mean silent—real strength is facing anxiety head-on."

Anxiety doesn't make you weak—it makes you human. **Overcoming Anxiety as a Man** offers practical tools, personal stories, and guided exercises to help you reframe negative thoughts, embrace vulnerability, and build resilience. This is more than a book—it's a companion for turning anxiety into strength and confidence.

### About the Author

Adam El-Asmer has faced anxiety since childhood, learning firsthand what it means to struggle in silence while searching for strength. Over the years, he's discovered how vulnerability, resilience, and self-reflection can transform anxiety into growth. Through sharing his story, Adam offers men a reminder that they are not alone and that every challenge can be a stepping stone toward confidence, purpose, and mental clarity.

ISBN 979-8-218-80748-1

www.ingramcontent.com/pod-product-compliance
Lightning Source LLC
Chambersburg PA
CBHW060142150626
46550CB00015B/2581